Gua Sha

Complete Natural Ways of Prevention and Treatment through Traditional Chinese Medicine to Maintain Perfect Health

Regina Williams

Table of Contents

GUA SHA 1

INTRODUCTION 5

CHAPTER 1 8
    WHAT ARE THE ADVANTAGES OF GUA-SHA? 8
        Will Gua-sha have Side Effects? 12

CHAPTER 2 14
    WHAT IS FACE GUA SHA? 14
    GREAT THINGS ABOUT GUA-SHA 15
        How to Perform Gua-Sha at Home 17
        Why is Lymphatic Drainage Important? 18

CHAPTER 3 23
    GUA-SHA MATERIALS: COMPREHENSIVE 23
    GUA SHA JADE STONE 26
    KONJAC FACE SPONGE - PURE 27
        Konjac Face Sponge - Bamboo Charcoal 28
        Konjac Face Sponge - Green Tea Extract 29
        Konjac Face Sponge - People from France Pink Clay 30

CHAPTER 4 33
    USES OF GUA-SHA 33
    BENEFITS 34
        Unwanted Effects and Risks 35
        Is Gua-sha painful? 37

CHAPTER 5 39
    HOW TO DO GUA-SHA FOR FACE IN 11 SIMPLE ACTIONS 39
    BENEFITS OF FACE GUA-SHA 39
    HOW IT WORKS 40

CHAPTER 6 45

How to Give Yourself the Best Gua-Sha Face at Home 45
How do you choose a Gua-sha Tool? 47
    How do you perform Gua-sha? 50
    How often must I practice Gua-sha? 54

CHAPTER 7 56

Beauty Restored - The Advantages of Face Gua-Sha 56

CHAPTER 8 60

CELLULITE 60
Body Acupuncture Treatment 61
    Gua-Sha Therapeutic massage Cellulite Singapore 65

CHAPTER 9 68

Gua-Sha: The DIY Beauty Tool for An Inside-Out Glow 68
Why Should We Make Dry Body Cleaning a Regular Habit 69
Can A Reiki Face Heal Your Skin Layer? 70

Copyright © 2020 by Regina Williams

All rights reserved. No part of this publication may be reproduced, distributed, or transmitted in any form or by any means, including photocopying, recording, or other electronic or mechanical methods, without the prior written permission of the publisher, except in the case of brief quotations embodied in critical reviews and certain other non-commercial uses permitted by copyright law.

ISBN: 978-1-63750-197-9

Introduction

Do you know that this ancient Chinese curing technique provides a unique method of better health and also dealing with issues like chronic pain.

Gua-sha is a part of traditional Chinese medication (TCM); it can also be known as "scraping," "spooning," or "coining." Its professionally use as an instrument to scrape people's pores and skin, it is said to have a therapeutic advantage. The procedure of this particular medication has a French name called *tribo-effleurage*. Gua-sha is an all-natural option therapy that involves scraping your skin layer with a therapeutic massage tool to boost your blood circulation.

Gua-sha is usually performed on the back, buttocks, neck, hands, and legs; a mild version from it is even applied to the facial skin as a cosmetic technique. Your specialist may apply moderate pressure, and steadily increase strength to regulate how much pressure you are designed for.

In gua-sha, a technician scrapes your skin layer with brief or long strokes to stimulate microcirculation of the smooth cells, which increases blood circulation; they make these strokes with a smooth-edged device known as a *Gua-therapeutic massage tool*, the specialist applies massage essential oil to your skin layer, and then uses the tool to scrape your skin layer in a downward movement frequently. Gua-sha is supposed to handle stagnant energy, called **chi**; professionals believe that this **"chi"** is responsible for swellings in any part of the body; swelling is the reason behind several conditions associated with chronic pain. Massaging the skin's surface is considered to help split up this energy, reduce irritation, and promote recovery.

Chapter 1

What are the Advantages of Gua-Sha?

Gua-sha may reduce swelling, so it's often used to take care of illnesses that cause chronic pain, such as ***arthritis and fibromyalgia***, as well as the ones that result in muscle and joint pain.

Gua-sha could also relieve symptoms of other conditions like:

1. *<u>Hepatitis B</u>*

Hepatitis B is a viral contamination that causes liver organ inflammation, liver harm, and liver organ scarring. Research shows that gua-sha may reduce persistent liver inflammation.

A trusted case study followed up a guy with high liver enzymes, an indication of liver irritation; he was presented with gua-sha medication, and after 48 hours of treatment, he experienced a decrease in liver organ enzymes. However, some experts also think that gua-sha can improve liver swelling, thus decreasing the probability of liver harm. More research is underway.

2. *Migraine headaches*

If your migraines do not relieve you after taking "over-the-counter medications," gua-sha can help. A study from a trusted source shows that a 72-year-old female coping with chronic headaches received gua-sha more than 14 days, and her migraine headaches relieved during this period, suggesting that the ancient curing technique may be a highly effective remedy for problems.

3. *Breast engorgement*

Breast engorgement is a disorder experienced by many breastfeeding women, i.e., when the chest is overfilled with dairy, this usually occurs in the first weeks of breastfeeding. The mother's breast becomes inflamed and painful, which makes it difficult for infants to latch. However, this usually is a short-term condition.

Study shows that women receive gua-sha from the next day after having a baby up until departing the hospital; a healthcare facility adopted the gua-sha medication on ladies in the weeks after having a baby, and they discovered that much-experienced relief of engorgement, breasts fullness, and pain, this made it easier for them to breastfeed.

4. *Neck pain*

Gua-sha technique has also been proved to be a very effective remedy for chronic throat pain. To look for the effectiveness of therapy, 48 research participants were put into two organizations; one group was presented with gua-sha, and the other used a thermal heating system pad to take care of throat pain. After seven days, individuals who received gua-sha reported less pain than the group that didn't receive gua-sha.

5. *Tourette syndrome*

Tourette symptoms involve ***involuntary motions*** such as face tics, neck clearing, and vocal outbursts. Relating to an individual, gua-sha coupled with other therapies may have helped to lessen symptoms of Tourette in the analysis participant.

The analysis involved a 33-year-old male who had Tourette syndrome at the age of 9; he received acupuncture, natural herbs, gua-sha, and altered his lifestyle, his symptoms relieved by 70 percent. Even though this man got excellent results, further research is necessary.

6. *Premenopausal syndrome*

Pre-menopausal occurs as women close to menopause. Medical indications include:

- Insomnia.

- Irregular periods.

- Anxiety.

- Fatigue.

- hot flashes

Studies, however, show that gua-sha may reduce premenopausal symptoms in a few women. The analysis examined 80 women with premenopausal symptoms. The treatment group received 15 tiny gua-sha treatments once weekly, together with standard therapy for eight weeks. The control group only received regular therapy.

Upon completion of the analysis, the involvement group reported a higher reduced amount of symptoms such as insomnia, anxiety, exhaustion, headaches, and hot flashes than the control group.

Experts believe gua-sha therapy might be considered a safe, effective treatment for these symptoms.

Will Gua-sha have Side Effects?

As an all-natural healing treatment, gua-sha is safe. It's not said to be unpleasant, but the process may change the looks of your skin layer because it entails massaging or scraping epidermis with a therapeutic massage tool, tiny arteries known as capillaries close to the surface of your skin layer can burst; this may result in pores and skin bruising and small blood loss. Bruising usually disappears within a few days.

Some individuals also experience short-term indentation

of their epidermis after a gua-sha treatment. Three necessary precautions will be listed below:

- If any bleeding occurs, there's also the chance of transferring blood-borne illnesses with gua-sha therapy, so technicians must disinfect their tools after every person.

- Avoid this system if you've acquired any surgery within the last six weeks.

- Folks who are taking bloodstream thinners or have clotting disorders aren't suitable applicants for gua-sha.

Chapter 2

What is Face Gua Sha?

Face Gua-Sha can be a well-known scraping massage technique produced by Traditional Chinese Medicine; it started as a cure done solely on your body to improve blood flow, move lymphatic stagnation, and releases muscle tension.

As time passes, a much gentler version was made for the facial skin, which involves a light gliding motion tone, lift, and smooths your skin. Tools of varied shapes manufactured from crystal (such as jade or Rose quartz) are used in combination with light pressure within an upward and outward movement.

The goal is to de-puff the facial skin by facilitating lymphatic drainage into the neck and bring fresh blood & nutrients to your skin for the healthy glow. As you gently scrape your skin, micro-circulation is improved, which carries oxygenated bloodstream to the dermal layers clearing congestion, stimulating cell renewal, and brightening your appearance. This hurry of blood brings nutrients that produce cell regeneration and tissues repair a lot more productive, which is incredibly helpful if you're dealing with acne or attempting to eliminate acne scars.

Overall, it's a remarkably easy addition to your morning hours or evening pores and skin routine that calls for 5 minutes and can offer you a noticeable lift and shine each time.

Gua-Sha Tools

Long-time ago, Gua-Sha scraping tools were manufactured from things such as bone or even cow horns. I used to be once told that is basically because cow horns are great conductors of energy, as cows use their horns to communicate; whether that's true or not, I have no idea, although I'd love to have confidence in the concept of telepathic cows. Irrespective, it seems sensible that crystals are used today because they are also thought to emit energy.

Great Things About Gua-Sha

Cosmetic Gua-Sha movement is a lymphatic liquid that gets built-up in the facial skin, which bears away poisons that can donate to acne and boring, irritated skin.

Gua-Sha benefits include:

- Shades the muscles of the facial skin which can help with sagging skin

- Companies and hydrates your skin

- Relaxes muscle stress in the facial skin, adding to full body stress alleviation (puts your body in a parasympathetic condition, which is wonderful for anybody that has trouble drifting off to sleep)

- Boosts blood circulation & circulation

- Moves stagnant bloodstream that plays a part in dark circles & under-eye bags.

- Helps your skin get over blemishes & acne scarring

- Prevents lines and wrinkles and helps clean existing lines

- De-puffs and slims the facial skin

- Instantly lifts and plumps your skin

- Allows serums to penetrate deeper post-treatment

- Aids throat pain & headaches due to tight muscle or fascia

How to Perform Gua-Sha at Home

If you want to begin at the throat/jaw first and work the right path up, so you start lymphatic drainage at the cheapest point; that way, when you get yourself up to your forehead and vision area, the liquid and poisons have someplace to drain into just like a funnel.

Additionally, you want to use very light pressure; if your skin layer begins to get very red, it's to company and not focusing on the lymph. Lymph needs light weight because your lymphatic vessels are so near to the top. Your tools should be angled at about 15-20°, almost smooth to your skin so that you're not stabbing yourself and can feel the soft pull that plays a part in the lifting impact.

Always scrape towards the outer sides of the facial skin and sweep down for the center when you're doing all your neck, which means that your lymph drains appropriately into the nodes above your collarbone.

Why is Lymphatic Drainage Important?

Did you know your lymphatic system is doubly significant as your circulatory system? While your circulatory system has your center to pump and clean your bloodstream automatically, your lymph does not have any built-in pump whatsoever. Lymph only goes by hand through exercise, therapeutic massage, and diet, which explains why it's straightforward to get supported by this modern lifestyle.

The lymphatic system had not been fully understood under western culture until less than two decades ago - yet ancient systems of medicine such as TCM or Ayurveda view is among the first places to consider stagnation when your body is ill. The AMA historically ignores lymph stagnation as a reason behind disease, whereas other countries such as Germany use specific

Lymphatic Drainage techniques as a cure for fibrocystic breast disease, allergies, persistent sinusitis, arthritis, eczema, cardiovascular disease and more.

An indicator that your lymphatic system is sluggish is:

- <u>If the body is a residence, think of your blood as the faucet as well as your lymph as the drains:</u> As I said, your bloodstream is always pumping, which means that your valves are continually operating. The problem is that they run directly into the area that isn't still assured to go. When waste materials particles from the bloodstream are too big to be removed by your liver organ, kidneys, or epidermis, it goes directly into your lymphatic vessels. So when those "drains" aren't moving correctly, stagnation and disease occur.

The most frequent factors behind poor lymphatic circulation are:

- **Stress** - The chemistry of stress is degenerative and lymph-congesting in character. Overwork and insufficient rest periods bargain your lymph, digestive function, and liver organ Qi.

- **Digestive Imbalances** - Irritation of the intestinal villi credited to inflammatory foods and poor digestion congests us because nearly all your lymph surrounds the gut via "Gut Associated Lymph Tissue" (GALT). See my post here about 11 uncommon (yet straightforward) ways to boost your digestion. To get more in-depth solutions, I've another post here that clarifies the four main factors behind poor digestion and exactly how to address all of them.

- **Deficiencies** - Nutrient deficiencies, especially iodine, impact the lymph. Iodine helps to mitigate the consequences of a harmful environment (hello pesticide-sprayed world!) and supports the lymph at a mobile level. See my post here on the advantages of seaweed.

- **Emotional/Religious** - Shame, blocked circulation of pleasure in life, depression, repressed emotions.

- **Insufficient Activity** - Since I explained that the

lymph does not have any pump, it depends on you to do it; an inactive lifestyle/working a table job seriously compromises lymphatic flow.

- **Diet** - Foods can either help or prevent the stream of lymph. Most severe: prepared/packaged, refined sugars (corn syrup), bleached flour.

Face Gua-Sha is one small area of the lymphatic puzzle, but it can certainly help to get things moving, particularly if you have chronic problems with mucus build-up in your sinuses.

Actions you can take to boost lymphatic blood circulation include:

- Take strolls daily, especially after foods (even for 10 minutes).

- Eat the white area of the orange! (click that for my post on this issue).

- Consume red-staining foods (pure cranberry juice, blueberries, and raspberries).

- Decrease the timeframe that you sit down per day

give dry-brushing a join a rebounder for only a few minutes, several times per day.

Chapter 3

Gua-Sha Materials: Comprehensive

Have a look at our list below so you can see the best materials to consider:

1. Bian Stone

Bian stones are believed to be the best tools for gua-sha because they have the most ultrasonic pulses and the best selection of frequency. The usage of Bian stones for therapeutic is centuries-old. In the *"Nei Jing,"* a historical Chinese Medical publication, it lists "acupuncture, moxibustion, natural medication, Qigong, and Bian rock therapy" as the five primary medical methods of the "Yellow Emperor," a deity in Chinese religious beliefs. What's impressive is that Bian rock therapy predates acupuncture.

If you wish to do Gua-Sha the authentic way, use Bian rocks.

2. Jade

Jade is our second best pick for gua-sha devices. It is stated to have qi energy that is nearly the same as the qi energy of the body. Therefore, it is perfect for healing treatments. In the olden times, barefoot doctors in China cannot afford traditional gua-sha tools, so they got scraps from jade carvers and used them as gua-sha tools. Today, jade continues to be widely used because of this healing technique.

3. Buffalo Horn

Genuine Bian rocks result from the town of *Sibin* in China. If you're struggling to find Bian rocks to use, Buffalo horn is another excellent option.

In Chinese medicine, a buffalo horn has a chilly property and an acrid/salty flavor. The acridity enhances qi and blood flow, nourishes, and moistens. The saltiness, on the other hand, relaxes tightness and softens hardness. Finally, the coldness dispels warmth and eliminates toxins in the torso.

While American buffalo are from the endangered list; if you worry about where buffalo horns result from getting jade, natural stone, or steel instead.

4. *Stainless Steel*

Medical-grade stainless tools are a favorite choice for *DASCM* (Device Assisted Soft Cells Mobilization) and are merely a modern development of Gua-Sha. If you'd like newer materials, you can consider Stainless or even Titanium implements.

5. *Rose Quartz*

Rose quartz is thought to open up the center chakra and reduce pressure in the center. It is a lovely stone which will come in a delicate red color.

Like a Gua-Sha tool, it is smooth and a good weight; others though think it is hard to hold and choose the buffalo horn or bian rock. Any object - just like a coin, a spoon, or a cover - can be utilized for Gua-Sha. Obtaining the best put into action, though, makes the complete experience convenient and, in ways, more memorable as you use tools that become special for you.

Using this method of an ancient form of recovery, you'll be managing your stress and diseases in more natural ways rather than counting on pharmaceuticals or even more vices that only bring short-term alleviation.

Gua Sha Jade Stone

Gua-Sha for the facial skin and neck is named the Eastern Botox or Eastern Facelift for grounds; this Traditional Chinese medication treatment, when put on the face, gets the following results:

- *Companies up your sagging face muscles*

- *Smoothens your skin and reduces the looks of lines and wrinkles on that person*

- *Improves dark circles and handbags under the eye (the type you get from advancing age group)*

- *Lightens age places and other pores and skin discolorations*

- *Your tone gets rosier and more radiant*

- *Helps get rid of acne, rosacea, and other epidermis diseases on that person.*

How exactly to use:

Our Rose Quartz Gua-Sha tools feature a printed beginner's guide to getting the most from it at home.

Konjac Face Sponge - Pure

Ideal for everyone, a 100% Pure Konjac Sponge deeply cleanses, gets rid of blackheads and gently exfoliates your skin. The unique online like framework of the veggie fibers helps to stimulate blood circulation and promote pores and skin cell renewal.

How exactly to use:

Before use, always wash the sponge thoroughly. We recommend plunging it in drinking water and squeezing it many times. If the sponge has dry out, ever let it fully absorb water before putting it against your skin layer.

Gently massage the facial skin and body in a circular motion around to exfoliate dead skin cells and deep cleanse. The massaging will stimulate exhausted epidermis & encourage pores and skin renewal. Soap or cleansing solution can be put into the sponge if desired but is not essential.

Your sponge should last almost a year, but once it begins to look tired, or begins to breakdown. Please replace it. The better treatment you take of your sponge, the much longer it'll last.

Konjac Face Sponge - Bamboo Charcoal

Packed with nutrient-rich triggered carbon, the Konjac Sponge with Bamboo Charcoal deep cleans pores to remove blackheads and dirt and grime while absorbing extra oils and toxins. An all-natural antioxidant, it kills persistent acne-causing bacteria, and it is a highly effective natural treatment for acne victims.

How exactly to use:

Before use, always wash the sponge thoroughly. We recommend plunging it in drinking water and squeezing it many times. If the sponge has dry out, ever let it fully absorb water before putting it against your skin layer.

Gently massage the facial skin and body in a circular motion around, to exfoliate dead skin cells, and deeply cleanse; the massaging will stimulate exhausted epidermis & encourage pores and skin renewal.s Soap or cleansing solution can be put into the sponge if desired but is not essential.

Your sponge should last almost a year, but once it begins to look tired, or begins to breakdown. Please replace it. The better treatment you take of your sponge, the much longer it'll last.

Konjac Face Sponge - Green Tea Extract

Green Tea herb is naturally filled with antioxidants that have a cell-protecting function; they have a substantial antioxidant impact that protects your skin from the damaging aftereffect of free radicals. This natural component has a softening and plumping effect on boosting elasticity and refreshing your skin's appearance, which is suitable for individuals who desire to protect the epidermis from aging.

How exactly to use:

Before use, always wash the sponge thoroughly. We recommend plunging it in drinking water and squeezing it many times. If the sponge has dry out, always let it fully absorb water before putting it against your skin layer.

Gently massage the facial skin and body in a circular motion around, to exfoliate dead skin cells, and deep cleanse. The massaging will stimulate exhausted pores and skin & encourage epidermis renewal. Soap or cleansing solution can be put into the sponge if desired but is not essential.

Your sponge should last almost a year, but once it begins to look tired, or begins to breakdown. Please replace it. The better treatment you take of your sponge, the much longer it'll last.

Konjac Face Sponge - People from France Pink Clay

The perfect Konjac Sponge for those experiencing the extremes of the elements of air-con, excess sun exposure, and central heating. Pure French Red Clay softly purifies even the most delicate pores and skin and has a softening and plumping impact on boosting elasticity and refreshing your skin's appearance.

How exactly to use:

Before use, always wash the sponge thoroughly. We recommend plunging it in drinking water and squeezing it many times. If the sponge has dry out, always let it fully absorb water before putting it against your skin layer.

Gently massage the facial skin and body in a circular motion around, to exfoliate dead skin cells, and deep cleanse. The massaging will stimulate exhausted epidermis & encourage pores and skin renewal. Soap or cleansing solution can be put into the sponge if desired but is not essential.

Your sponge should last almost a year, but once it begins to look tired, or begins to breakdown. Please replace it. The better treatment you take of your sponge, the much longer it'll last.

Konjac Face Sponge - Lavender

Lavender is an all-natural relaxant and detoxifier with

impressive recovery capabilities. This beautiful blossom has strong skills to relaxed and reduces stress and anxious tension, which makes it ideal for soothing skin treatment.

How exactly to use:

Before use, always wash the sponge thoroughly. We recommend plunging it in drinking water and squeezing it many times. If the sponge has dry out, always let it fully absorb water before putting it against your skin layer.

Gently massage the facial skin and body in a circular motion around to exfoliate dead skin cells and deep cleanse. The massaging will stimulate exhausted epidermis & encourage pores and skin renewal. Soap or cleansing solution can be put into the sponge if desired but is not essential.

Your sponge should last almost a year, but once it begins to look tired, or begins to breakdown. Please replace it. The better treatment you take of your sponge, the much longer it'll last.

Chapter 4
Uses of Gua-sha

Listed below are various methods of gua-sha meditation technique:

- Gua-sha is frequently used to alleviate muscle and joint pain; conditions of the muscles and bone fragments are known as musculoskeletal disorders, a few examples include back pain, tendon stress, and carpal tunnel symptoms.

- Practitioners declare that gua-sha also has the advantage of disease-fighting capability and reduction of irritation. Sometimes, gua-sha is utilized to take care of a chilly, fever, or issues with the lungs.

- Small injuries to your body, like the bruises caused by gua-sha, are occasionally known as micro-trauma; these create a reply in the torso that might help to split up scar tissue. Micro-trauma also may help with fibrosis, which is an accumulation of too much connective tissue when your body heals.

- Physiotherapists could use IASTM on connective cells that are not attempting to move bones as it will; this issue may be credited to repetitive stress damage or another condition. Gua-sha can be used alongside other treatments, such as extending and conditioning exercises.

Benefits

Researchers have completed small studies on the next groups of individuals to find out if gua-sha works:

- Women close to menopause.

- People with the neck of the guitar and make pain from computer use.

- Male weightlifters, to assist with recovery after training.

- Old adults with back pain.

- Women discovered that pre-menopausal symptoms,

such as perspiration, insomnia, and headaches were reduced after gua-sha.

A 2014 study discovered that gua-sha improved the number of motion and reduced pain in people who use computer systems frequently. Also, anther research in 2017 shows that weightlifters that had gua-sha experienced found it easier to lift weight after treatment.

Old adults with back pain were treated with either gua-sha or a hot pack; both treatments relieved symptom similarly well; however, the ramifications of gua-sha lasted much longer. After weekly, those who ha received gua-sha treatment reported greater versatili and less back pain than the other group.

Unwanted Effects and Risks

Gua-sha often burst tiny arteries close to the surface your skin called *capillaries*. It creates the distinctive r or crimson bruises, known as *sha*. The injuries usual take a couple of days or weekly to heal and can be tend while healing, people may take an over-the-coun painkiller, such as ibuprofen, to assist with pain a oating. A person should protect the bruised area mindful never of bumping it (applying a ⟨ can help reduce swelling and simplicity any

professionals shouldn't break your skin through lent, but there's a risk it might happen; broken surface increases the probability of illness, so a pecialist should sterilize their tools between

s not ideal for everybody; individuals who lave gua-sha include those:

) have medical ailments affecting your skin or s?

bleed easily.

take medication to thin their blood.

've deep vein thrombosis?

have contamination, tumor, or wound that healed fully.

se quartz. Medical quality stainless is often used for STM or when gua-sha is performed in a medical center. ofessionals will apply essential oil to the region of your dy that has been treated, which allows the therapist to e the tool over the epidermis more smoothly. The gua-a practitioner will press the device into the body with 100th, firm strokes in a single path; if Gua-sha has been mpleted on the trunk or back of the legs, a person ight need to lay face down on a therapeutic massage ble.

- Who has an implant, like a pacemaker defibrillator.

Is Gua-sha painful?

Treatment is not said to be painful, b deliberately causes bruising, which mi discomfort for a lot of people; these bruises in a few days.

Gua-Sha Tools and Techniqu

Gua-sha equipment

A handheld tool with curved edges is utilized Typically, a spoon or coin would be employe your skin; however, in modern practice, ther little, hand-held tool with rounded edges.

Gua-sha tools tend to be weighted to help th doing the task to use pressure.

Professionals of traditional East Asian mec some materials as having a power that v recovery - these materials include bian-rock

Chapter 5

How to do Gua-Sha for Face in 11 Simple Actions

Once I first noticed you might have a Gua-Sha for face and throat, I had been amazed. I've been a lover of this historic treatment but didn't realize that there is a face version.

Benefits of Face Gua-Sha

Gua-Sha, for the facial skin and neck, is named the *Eastern Botox (or Eastern Facelift)*. This traditional Chinese medication treatment, when put on the face, gets the following results:

- Help your sagging facial muscles.

- Smoothens your skin and reduces the looks of lines and wrinkles on that person.

- Improves dark circles and handbags under the eye (the type you get from advancing age group).

- Lightens age and other pores and skin discolorations.

- Your tone gets rosier and more radiant.

- Helps get rid of acne, rosacea, and other epidermis diseases on that person

I have a first-hand connection with everything on the list aside from the last, and even though I used to be expecting great results due to my positive encounters with body Gua-Sha, I had been still amazed to start to see the improvements on my face.

I'd halted taking Glutathione and Grape Seed, but after a couple of weeks of face Gua-Sha, my face has a clearness and radiance that I'd only as a rule have while on those supplements.

How it Works

As discussed above, Gua-Sha is identified to be the age-old practice that involves the scraping movements all around the surface of one's body with a smooth-edged tool; it is hard enough to improve petechial, reddish marks that typically transmit a Gua-Sha therapy program.

Gua-Sha scraping

Face Gua-Sha is a lot much milder but gets the same scraping action along your skin; as your skin is scraped, the layers of your skin are activated, and stagnant lymph that triggers puffiness is relocated and cleared from the system; poisons are also released, producing a brighter appearance and lastly, the massaging action relaxes anxious muscles that wrinkles provide.

Eastern Botox in 11 Steps

Several reminders for beginners:

- Don't use the same heavy pressure that you utilize when scraping your body. Because of this to work, you should employ only light weight. The facial skin is more delicate than other areas of your body.

- We are moving stagnant lymph from our face. We will drain this out via the right and remaining lymphatic ducts. They are the areas among your collarbones.

- All our (light) scraping movements will be upwards. Keep in mind; we are countering sagging, so we can't ever make any downward actions. The only exclusion is the finished part whenever we do the dumping in the lymphatic ducts highlighted above.

Cosmetic Gua-sha

Now here will be the general steps you can do as a newbie:

- <u>Third Vision</u>: Heart stroke from the center of your eyebrows or more to your hairline. This area activates curing.

- <u>Lower forehead</u>: Sweep from the guts of the forehead above your eyebrows venturing out to your temples.

- <u>Under eyebrow</u>: Utilize the curved part of your gua-sha tool to scrape the region underneath your eyebrow and above your eye. Stick to the bone of the brow.

- <u>Under the eye</u>: Slowly and lightly stroke the region where your vision bags typically show; begin from the medial side of your nasal area and rise to your temple. Imagine moving the stagnant lymph from the center of that person up to the temple and entirely to the hairline.

- <u>Cheek</u>: Do the same sweeping movement for the cheek area. Go from the medial side of your nasal area, across your cheek, or more again to the center of your ear.

- <u>Jaws</u>: Do the same for the jaws again, sweeping the lymph upwards to your ear.

- <u>Chin</u>: Sweep from the center of that person, under your lower lip, and also to the earlobe.

- <u>Under chin</u>: Scrape from the soft area under your chin to underneath of your hearing.

- <u>Throat</u>: Finally, it's time for you to scrape from

your jaw and earlobe right down to the center of your collarbone.

- <u>The best sweep</u>: Collect all the lymph you've moved aside of the facial skin and dumped it to your lymphatic drainage, sweep from the guts of your forehead right under your hairline, right down to your temple, right down to your hearing until you achieve your throat and terminus area. Do many times for a clean sweep.

Chapter 6

How to Give Yourself the Best Gua-Sha Face at Home

What exactly does gua-sha do?

Gua-sha pre-dates acupuncture; the heart stroke design used, awakens the meridian lines (life force route) to activate the body's natural curing abilities. For your skin, gua-sha stimulates collagen creation (power in cells); it sculpts and shades the face form, allowing irritation to drain and muscles to be free of pressure - permitting them to make their supportive careers properly. Also, it helps your skin go back to its most radiant condition as blood circulation is increased, sending nutrition to areas that might have been starved because of blockage.

Gua-Sha's impact is more than pores and skin deep; as the meridian lines are enlivened, organs like the belly, liver, spleen, center, and kidneys also receive a great advantage. Dealing with gua-sha tools over the region of the facial skin linked to the kidneys allows them to operate at ideal capacity.

What are the huge benefits?

- Bears nutrient-rich and oxygenated bloodstream (food for the cells) to your skin and tissues

- Drains lymph liquid (which is often filled up with toxins and waste materials) from the cells to be cleansed

- Eliminates or significantly reduces wrinkles

- Treats and helps prevent sagging epidermis (elevates and tightens your skin)

- Aids in removing dark circles around the eyes

- Aids in splitting up and liberating your skin from shaded areas and hyper-pigmentation

- Brightens the complexion

- Exceedingly rates of speed the curing time of breakouts and acne, helping these pores and skin issues overall

- Has the capacity to heal and relieve rosacea

- Supports product penetration

- Goodies TMJ disorder and migraines

- Is an alternative to shots and face-lift surgery (when used frequently at home or when getting treatments from a certified practitioner)

How do you choose a Gua-sha Tool?

Gua-sha tools come in an array of different designs, sizes and forms; some devices are produced from pet bone and horn, some from gemstones (like jade or increased quartz), plus some professionals use the Chinese soup spoons. I've even seen the cover of a cup jar (one with curved and soft sides) found in a pinch.

Trending right now is increased quartz and jade; jade is well known for inviting serenity and purity, as well as promoting fertility, balance, and deep recovery. Rose quartz is well known for restoring tranquillity deep into the heart. It's the stone of universal love and promotes unconditional caring and compassion.

Choosing your gua-sha rock is comparable to choosing a crystal or gemstone. If you're able to choose it out personally, please do this. Pick and choose it up, feel it, observe it feels in your hands. Notice which catches your attention - if the first is sparkling a bit more for you than others, choose it!

What's the key to a rewarding practice?

Regularity is the key; to keep up a flourishing and maintain a healthy body, we regularly nourish ourselves with drinking water, rest, clean eating, and motion. Likewise, training gua-sha frequently will prove most appropriate. Your body doesn't thrive whenever we are oscillating to either extreme - the center is always most appropriate.

Since there are 20 liters of liquid that circulate through your body every day (and around three liters of the fluid becomes lymph liquid), it's very supportive to your body to create this practice into the day to day routine. However, getting gua-sha into your daily life each day may be challenging, but carving out an excellent little time a couple of days weekly is active (even if it's only two minutes). You may notice the body beginning to crave these occasions of self-care.

Pressure and purpose are also crucial to your practice; the touch should be very soft, and you may experiment with different levels of pressure. But always sweep the gua-sha rock across that person in specific movements. The lighter the touches, the higher you are assisting the lymph liquid, and with an increase of pressure, know you're getting into muscle. Please be careful that you shouldn't bruise or cause distress.

How do you prep your skin?

Having a clean face and clean hands, mist generously with a hydrosol *(I like True Botanicals Renew Nutrient Mist, OSEA's Sea Vitamin Boost or Heritage Store's Rose Water),* then apply facial oil *(I like True Botanicals Renew Radiance Oil, OSEA's Undaria Argan Oil or Shiva Rose face oil)* around that person and neck; using the essential oil left on the hands, grease up your gua-sha tool. Then, start - all while taking deep, cleansing breaths.

How do you perform Gua-sha?

Cleanse Face and Hands - After drying out the facial skin with a clean washcloth, generously mist that person. The hydrosol is an excellent vehicle to operate a vehicle the essential oil - which you'll apply next - deep into the epidermis, especially to the layers that require nourishment and hydration. (Suggestion: I only use my washcloth once, and then it goes into the hamper. If you have problems with breakouts, it is best not to reuse cosmetic towels before cleaning. Bacteria can transfer back again onto your skin.)

Apply Facial - Essential oil (from 4-10 drops), within the face and throat; apply essential oil starting on the forehead and moving down in the direction of draining lymph liquid. This activates motion in pores and skin and cells, and it's a good prep before the gua-sha.

Warm Gua-Sha Tool - slightly by rubbing it in the middle of your hands. This also greases the tool up a little so that it doesn't draw on your skin layer in the areas that didn't receive as much essential oil.

Sweep Up Your Neck Of The Guitar On Both Edges - Sweep very softly over your Adam's apple; this is more of a quick sweep to activate your REN collection. (The REN route in Chinese medication collects the body's yin energy, goodies the issues of the stomach, chest, neck, mind, and face.)

Sweep Under Your Chin - from the center of your face away to your earlobe, maintaining your tool smooth. If you'd like, contain the epidermis under your chin with your other thumb as you glide the device back again to your earlobe on the contrary direction.

Sweep From The Centre Of Your Chin Over Your Jawline - back again toward your earlobe; you can gently jiggle at the hearing to encourage the liquid to drain down the throat to the lymph nodes at the bottom, just above your collarbone.

Sweep Underneath Your Cheekbone - really picking right up a great deal of liquid that is commonly stored here, and direct it toward your hairline. You can lightly and lightly jiggle your tool at the hairline.

Sweep over Your Cheekbones - finishing at the hairline.

Very Gently Sweep Under Your Eye - I like sweeping from the part of the attention relocating toward the midline; the muscle agreements in this path and the lymph has little streams moving down from the eye entirely from the internal corner of the attention to the outer part. But if it seems easier to sweep from the interior edge of the care to the hairline, and then do this - this is a far more traditional path for gua-sha.

Sweep On The Eyebrow Out Toward The Hairline Or More From Your Brow Bone - (in the forehead) finishing at the hairline; when you sweep up, get it done in tiny areas, moving along the eyebrow in 3 to 5 sections.

Sweep from Between your Eyebrows over the 3rd Eye or More to the Hairline - Notice if your clairvoyance seems more activated following this stroke

Sweep From The Centre Of The Forehead Out To The Hairline - Among my favorite techniques originates from *Britta Plug of Britta Beauty in NYC*. She sweeps from the center of the forehead and doesn't touch the hairline and proceeds into the locks, behind the hearing and down the throat. It feels divine.)

Now Caress the Other Part of that Person - starting again with your neck and working through the steps.

Slide Down The Medial Side - When you've completed the other aspect of that person, finish the procedure by sweeping down the throat to aid with enduring drainage. Keep the tool very toned and hug underneath your jawbone, gently sweep down the throat to the collarbone.

<u>Key tips to help make the majority of your practice:</u>

- I would recommend sweeping each area at minimal three times; for extended practice, sweep up to 10 times.

- Maintain your tool level to your skin layer (about 15 degrees) rather than getting the advantage of the tool at 90 degrees to your skin layer.

- Whenever your tool begins to pull or draw on your skin layer, put in a little more essential oil for a better slide.

- Have fun tinkering with which aspect and form of

the tool best suit that person. Keep in mind, what feels right for you, may look unique of how it appears in videos.

How often must I practice Gua-sha?

I would recommend incorporating gua-sha into the self-care routine daily, but when it begins to feel just like a task, have a break.

Precisely what will it feel just like?

Gua-sha is often referred to as very relaxing, mainly when the pressure is merely right, use adoring, and mild strokes; be intentional in your touch. It will feel like you are sweeping the gua-sha on the beautiful, soft skin of the baby.

You might feel the fluids moving, which is fantastic! You may even feel your skin layer becoming alive or as though it's returning and getting up. I often time start the medication from the still left, as it is said to be the medial side of the feminine energy, which is more utilized at receiving. I've pointed out that when the remaining team of that person gets, it primes the right part to become more responsive.

How much gua-sha is too much?

Avoid gua-sha if you merely received injections. *Botox* requires at least fourteen days staying.

Avoid gua-sha over cystic acne, pimples, and open up lesions, as it will only irritate contaminated areas, but gua-sha is very beneficial within the breakout. Draining below the breakout allows the lymph to transport poisons to the lymph nodes. That's where waste materials will be cleansed before the time for the circulatory system to nourish your body.

Repeat each heart stroke within the same area, not more than ten times. If you are repeating the sweeping too many times, you may cause too much activation. Liquids are potent; you could finish up moving too much waste materials at one time, causing detoxification symptoms (such as dizziness or emotions of decreasing with the flu).

Chapter 7

Beauty Restored - The Advantages of Face Gua-Sha

Transform your tone with these facial therapeutic massage techniques. You can tell a lot about someone by merely taking a look at their face, not only the manifestation of their pulling or the immediate feeling they are actually. But health and wellness are also written on that person, and that's because, according to Chinese medication, your beauty can be an external representation of your internal health.

So our beauty routines are definite improvements to your wellbeing. Our creator and resident physician, Katie, has captured the substance of a large number of many years of Chinese wisdom into some powerful one-minute rituals. Quick and straightforward to do, they can fit neatly into our modern lives, supplying a transformative method of health and wellness, subsequently giving you a wholesome, glowing, and radiant tone.

Bring back your beauty

We're going to show you three iconic Chinese approaches for improving your appearance, we've processed them, and that means they could be done in only about a minute each.

They are Àn-fa (press-hold) Gua-Sha (press stroke) and Acupressure (press-turn).

It's been found in the Chinese facial therapeutic massage for a large number of years and revered because of its restorative, chilling properties.

Our studies showed that 82% of women found an immediate, positive impact after just one minute of use.

- **Àn-fa**

In this system, you need to press and contain the *jade Beauty RestorerTM* over that person; press-holding the jade may reduce swelling and increase lymphatic drainage.

You can take the wonder *RestorerTM* on the eyes to alleviate fatigue, alleviate eyesight bags, puffy eye, or twitching eyes muscles. You can even use the jade tool over any area to ease stress-related symptoms such as headaches, flushing, pores and skin conditions, and throbbing temples.

- **Gua-Sha**

Gua-Sha is a straightforward press and heart stroke technique along the curves of that person, as shown. This beauty treatment has been used across Asia for a large number of years. It's renowned because of its unique capability to increase blood flow under your skin, bringing in nutrition and improving collagen.

So, rather than applying a cream or serum to boost your skin layer from the exterior, you're activating the body to nourish your skin layer in a far more profound and meaningful way. This self-massage technique has been proven in studies to improve circulation by 400%. It stimulates the dermis to aid collagen creation, manipulating regions of stress to relax cosmetic muscles, exponentially raises bloodstream and lymphatic movement. All of this leads to a brighter, healthier, more radiant tone.

- **Acupressure**

Activating acupressure factors on that person is a superb way to aid your organs internally. Chinese medication recognizes that cosmetic beauty is from the organs in this manner - the condition of your wellbeing shown in that person.

Chapter 8

CELLULITE

Cellulite usually starts around the hips and thighs and mostly along the yang meridians; the starting place is often the Gall Bladder, the smaller yang meridian, perhaps because the Qi in the Gall Bladder is significantly less than in the other yang meridians. Cellulite explains the dimpling of your skin, triggered by the protrusion of subcutaneous excess fat into the dermis, creating an undulating junction between your pores and skin and subcutaneous adipose cells.

The Spleen nourishes muscle and fat, and the function of the Spleen is to distribute fat evenly through your body, especially in the periphery. Regarding cellulite, the extra fat distribution is affected, and fat appears to stagnate without circulation in some regions of the body. So, on the main one hand, there is undoubtedly extra fat, and on the other, there is undoubtedly poor circulation from it. This creates the picture of imbalance explained above.

However, we likewise have the problem in the meridian along which this issue occurs - that could be Gall Bladder but can also be Urinary Bladder or even Stomach, concerning the patient. So both Spleen and the affected meridians have to be well balanced.

Body Acupuncture Treatment

Example - cellulite on the lateral part of thighs

- Gall Bladder - UB 19 (Back-Shu point), GB 37 (Luo point).

- Spleen - UB 20 (Back-Shu point), St 40 (Luo point).

- Local needles and moving cup massage.

- Two sessions weekly, 8-10 sessions altogether.

This treatment principle can be utilized Atlanta divorce attorneys affected meridian. For instance, for the Bladder meridian - you can use UB 28 (the Back-Shu point, to enhance the function) and UB 58 (the Luo-connecting point of yang meridian, to tonify the yang and decrease the yin aspect).

Local treatment is quite useful if performed well. Patients sometimes want to hurry through the local procedure because cupping therapeutic massage is not so pleasant - it's essential to be patient while taking this treatment.

Special local therapy

If the affected area is privately along the Gall Bladder meridian, this treatment should be achieved in two halves, with the individual lying using one side first and having all the fine needles and cupping; then fired up the other aspect and getting the same treatment.

- Lying privately, points on your body - UB 18, UB 20, St 40, GB 37.

- At precisely the same time, about 10 to 15 local fine needles in the region of the cellulite (15-20 cm fine needles of 0.20 mm gauge) are inserted wholly and perpendicularly, at about 3 cm distance from one another.

- Both body needles and local needles are remaining in situ for 20 minutes.

- After all of the needles are removed, apply *St John's wort* oil sparingly on the region of cellulite. Usually, do not overdo this, as it'll reduce friction for the therapeutic massage.

- Place a big cup (for a particular cellulite glass) at the low end of the thigh using an open fire for creating vacuum pressure, and slip the container along the region until the epidermis becomes quite red. This process is quite unpleasant for the individual, and if very sore, then your vacuum could be reduced. The therapeutic massage takes about a minute.

- The individual may remark that the legs feel very light following the treatment.

- Treatment is administered twice regularly, for 8-10 times as a course.

What can the individual do at home?

As cellulite is stagnation of fat, the individual can do a lot of things at home to avoid its formation and also to improve circulation.

- Foods that induce fat tissue in the torso are; fatty foods, fatty dairy food (low-fat dairy food can be consumed in small amounts), refined sugars, and sugar (though wholemeal, fruits, sugars, and honey are fine). These food types should be avoided.

- When fat tissue becomes too thicker, the blood circulation is affected. It is, therefore, important that the individual drinks drinking water regularly and during the day - the regularity is more important than the number consumed. Tepid to warm water is preferable to cool, which is impressive how quickly patients come to enjoying tepid to warm water.

- Finally, they ought to work daily in the region of the cellulite, massaging it with very soft spiky toners and pummelling these areas to break the stagnation. Seated cross-legged on to the floor and moving sideways and ahead and back this position, leading to friction on regions of cellulite ('bum walking'), for quarter-hour each day in the comfort of their house can be an additional solution to help improve blood circulation flow.

Gua-Sha Therapeutic massage Cellulite Singapore

Are you searching for a treatment for the unequal, lumpy pores and skin on your hips, thighs, or buttocks? The Gua-Sha Therapeutic massage Cellulite brings everything to the desk; you don't have to be ashamed of your body appearance any longer.

- Meet Gua-Sha: The Cellulite Remover

Gua-Sha therapeutic massage is a therapy technique used to take care of several ailments; included in these are aches and pains, strains, lumbar stress, arthritis rheumatoid, and heat heart stroke. The activation of blood circulation triggers its therapeutic impact; this relieves bloodstream stagnation. Moreover, the Gua-Sha Massage Cellulite gets rid of or reduces the introduction of cellulite in the torso.

Great things about Gua-Sha:

- Improves hydration levels.

- Relieves stress.

- Gets rid of or reduces Cellulite.

- Relaxes face muscles.

- Improves blood circulation etc.

Gua-Sha Therapeutic Massage Treatment:

Your skin is oily, and a Gua-Sha device is gently used to scrape over the surface of the affected area; this promotes breakage of surface adhesion, increases circulation, and enhances lymph drainage and firmness; it also solves the problems of fats cells and encourages a smoother appearance. Gua-Sha can be carried out on any area of the body. It could be performed in every area of the body, even on the facial skin. It can help to relax your skin and enhance the blood circulation flow in the facial skin and improve collagen creation; it gets your skin layer look more radiant and reduces lines and wrinkles.

Also, people utilize massage techniques or dry brushing to eliminate cellulite. The triggering of cells manually helps to improve blood circulation and also reduces adipose tissue, specifically in keeping energies like unwanted fat. Thus, it boosts skin radiance.

Chapter 9

Gua-Sha: The DIY Beauty Tool for An Inside-Out Glow

Self-care and skincare appear to go together; *Eva Ramirez* explores the historic ritual of Gua-sha and exactly how it can promote health insurance and radiance from within.

PAMELA HANSON

Gua-sha (pronounced gwa-sha) can be an old self-care practice found in traditional Chinese medicine when a tool, usually created from jade, bone or horn, is scraped over the epidermis to redirect energy stream. By doing this, stagnant energy is divided, reducing irritation, increasing blood circulation, and stimulating the lymphatic system to market healing in the torso. It's a straightforward but demanding technique that is used for years and years to treat problems such as fever, muscle pain, and pressure, swelling, chronic coughs, sinusitis, and migraine headaches.

Self-care is a center point of Chinese medication, where it is recognized as Yang Sheng (healthy life), and traditionally, Gua-sha was practiced at home. As is just how with many historic wellness customs, it's become ever more popular under western culture. Much like cupping or acupressure, many acupuncturists and professionals offer Gua-sha therapeutic massage as a cure in their treatment centers. Like a sports activities massage therapy, but with a prop, it is conducted with medium to extreme pressure around a person's back again, neck, legs, and arms, honing in on whichever areas specifically need of attention. The friction from the repeated strokes leads to scary-looking bruising and inflammation that can last for times after treatment.

Why Should We Make Dry Body Cleaning a Regular Habit

What exactly does this have to do with beauty and skincare? Well, a gentler version of the Gua-sha technique works like a miracle when applied on the facial skin. There's no need to visit a therapist because everything, as regards your skin, has been taken care of through your regular everyday skincare.

Can A Reiki Face Heal Your Skin Layer?

All you need is a Gua-sha tool, and about a minute each day to see instantaneous results and long-term benefits. Studies show that daily ritual enhances microcirculation by up to 400%, reduces wrinkles, rejuvenates, tones and smooths skin, boosts collagen, combats pigmentation, dark circles, and puffy eyes, defines jawlines and even decongests the sinuses. It's literally like rubbing the right path to healthier, glower skin. Since it primarily works from the within out, you'll also notice a release of tension and relaxing of facial muscles, if you clench your jaw during the night it's a terrific way to ease any soreness each day. If you often get eye twitches from insomnia or stress, holding the Gua-sha over your eyes with gentle pressure can also help relieve and relax the muscles.

To be sure you're using the right tools for the work, it's better to get a Gua-sha manufactured from jade. Apart from looking beautiful on your dresser, this green rock is revered because of its air conditioning properties; staying away from anything created from bone and horn for apparent reasons; it's also advisable to stay away from cheaper alternatives that could be produced from acrylic or other artificial substances that can irritate your skin. Applying facial oil before massaging can help the stone to glide easier while moisturizing your skin too.

Katie Brindle is a Chinese medicine specialist and creator of *Hayo'u*, an all-natural health insurance and skincare brand located in the United Kingdom. *Hayo'u* makes the self-treatment facet of Chinese medication accessible and approachable with simple daily rituals and useful techniques. They provide the various tools, such as their Gua-sha, which is carved from traditional *Xiuyan Jade* and includes a velvet pouch (perfect for traveling) as well as short easy-to-follow videos to be able to perfect the ritual at home.

Whether practiced is the very first thing to do as a morning hours ritual or as an evening wind-down to eliminate the day's stress from that person, this mindful beauty practice is meditative and relaxing.

www.ingramcontent.com/pod-product-compliance
Lightning Source LLC
Chambersburg PA
CBHW071123030426
42336CB00013BA/2188